I Will, I Am, I Was.

Jason Jean

DEDICATION

I want to dedicate this book to the individual, family and company that is going through a change and wondering if you can make. I'm here to tell you, you can and will!

CONTENTS

ACKNOWLEDGMENTS

I want to sincerely thank not only everyone who has ever stood by, but anyone who has gone through a life changing experience. Everybody defines life as their own journey…their own transcendence.

Outcomes and consequences of my life have equipped me to adjust, to be responsive and how to effectively reinvent myself. I'm not unique in my ability; I witness it every day from the waitress at my favorite restaurant that just lost her job to my best friends and colleagues. Reinvention is a necessity for growth and maturity…don't perceive it as a negative because anything that can empower you as an individual can be positively effective to the world around you.

Embrace those around you. Reinvention is not always about picking yourself up, it can also be about continuing to propel to the next level. Being multifaceted and accelerating forward through your life will aid in your strength of will and mind.

Experiences like enduring seven knee operations related to playing football, or surviving falling 22 feet allowed me to see life in a different way. Like many athletes, it's difficult, to say the least, to have to let go and even mourn something you always thought you would always be and accepting what you have become. When you are helplessly lying in a cold and blank hospital room, hurting more and trying to remember what day it was when you last saw your kids compared to the physical pain of surviving, it's a call of consciousness. During my recovery from a life-threatening fall, I looked at my wife and saw her strength and her great ability to be able to not only mend me back to health, but to take care of our young children and hold herself together, too.

This book is for everyone that has, or is going through a phenomenal life event, that wonders how or why they can get through one more stressor, one more minute. Believe that you can by reinventing the best thing you know-yourself. Have fortitude and perseverance. It's important to know how incredible life is and to love everything it has to offer.

INTRODUCTION

Did you ever aspire to do something or be someone extraordinary? Is there a voice or a barrier that makes you doubt your ability to succeed at the extraordinary?

Right now, I want to focus on your dreams, aspirations and goals in life. I want to help motivate you to reach specific goals, while keeping you and your expectations grounded. I want you to learn to be realistic about what you can truly achieve. It's important to note that being a realist does not diminish your achievements, great or small; being a realist should always be your motivation to conquer and reach for higher targets. Become clear with your barriers, make peace with them and isolate your obstacles.

Whether you are the next great athlete, world renowned chef, or the next big pop star, I want you to focus on what it takes mentally, emotionally and physically to achieve your goal or goals in some cases. I need you to look in the mirror and see the potential I see in you, if you are taking

1

the time to read this, YOU CAN MAKE IT! Surround yourself with great people that believe in you and who will support you through the ups and downs while you are on your path to success.

You need to realize how important it is to work hard from a young age to allow yourself all the opportunities available to you so you can cement your place in the world of greatness.

1 DREAMS VS. GOALS

As a child you made and achieved goals without realizing it because the process was simple and the goals were small in comparison to your goals later in life. You simply said to yourself that you were going to climb the backyard tree, maybe get a hit at your next baseball game or win at the 40 yard dash in grade school...then you set off to make it happen. The goals you set fit your age, your ability and eventually—without you even realizing it—propelled you forward, impacting what you do in the future.

But now, as you grow older, goals tend to have much more significance to you because they have more depth, longevity and meaning. Additionally, your goals may take longer to achieve, which means you may need to have patience while setting them.

Your goals and dreams are close in connotation, especially when they're close to your heart and convictions. The major difference between goals and dreams are obviously their definitions, but more importantly their end results.

3

Let's take a closer look.

Dream: a noun-*something hoped for: something that somebody hopes, longs, or is ambitious for, usually something difficult to attain or far removed from present circumstances and is an aspiration.* Example: "I want to play for the Yankees." This would be considered a dream because you dream that someday you'll play for the Yankees.

Now, let's see how you can take this dream and turn it into a goal.

Goal: a noun-*The purpose toward which an endeavor is directed; an objective; and the result or achievement toward which effort is directed; aim; end.*

Example: I will someday play in the majors.

I will talk later in the book about being a realist and talk about hurdles you just may not be able to get over to achieve your goal. I've taken your dream of playing for the Yankees and made your dream broader and turned it into an actual goal to make it in the majors. By doing this, you have an actual goal to work toward—one that is more obtainable. You can still dream of someday playing for the Yankees, realizing playing for a specific team in this case could be out of your control so you may never actually be able to make that dream into a goal or reality. There will be some goals in life you just can't obtain and that's okay, you will (later in the book) learn to adapt and adjust those goals.

When turning your dreams into goals, be aware of the difference. You'll have to ask yourself if this dream you are trying to turn into a goal is actually attainable. Let's look at an example:

You want to play a professional sport and you are twelve when you make this decision, I'd say it is a goal to work toward, because you are a kid and you can control your own destiny (to a certain point) but you will need to work toward that goal and at this point anything is possible. But and there is a but, if you are 19, 5'3, 100 pounds and you're done growing and you say you want to play professional football, you have to reexamine if that goal is still attainable. Maybe you'll have to adapt your goal to something that is obtainable. This will happen throughout your life; as I described above, there will be obstacles in certain professions when certain specifics are required. Perhaps a certain body size or a specific ability is crucial. Whatever it might be, if you don't meet that criteria there is a good chance you may need to adapt your goal. Don't look at this as a failure, because there are some things that are out of your control. Look at it as a positive…when you adapt and change goals, you get to reinvent yourself; you get to find new strengths within yourself that you might have never known you had.

Too often, people talk about their dreams but it seems they hardly mention their goals. Goals and dreams don't always have to be sports or career-oriented, they could be as simple as, I want to go on vacation, and I want to see the Washington Monument. Just like above, I know it's a simple play on words, but by changing the words to I will or I am going on vacation or I will or I am going to the Washington Monument changes things. But, it doesn't stop with a few words; there are other steps you need to take including setting dates for the vacation, getting time off work, etc. If it's a dream to do something someday, you need to take the steps to make it a reality. I know you may think this is a ridiculous example of a goal but, something as small as a vacation can and will be important at some point in your life. This will teach you that you can accomplish even the simplest goals.

Everyone has set a goal at some point in their lives that they didn't or will not achieve but, do they pay attention to why? One of the main reasons why some goals are not met is because in order to succeed, the goal setter needs to know the basics of setting the right goals while differentiating those goals from dreams, again obtainable goals.

Let me give you another example of how to turn a dream into a goal, I'm sure you know someone that knows someone that knows someone who has run a marathon, and I'm sure at some point you have said either, "boy, I wish I could run one" or "man, I could never run one." If you are the one who would love to try it but doesn't feel you could do it and who just keeps saying, "I want to run in a marathon," or "I wish I could run in a marathon," it will always just be a dream. You don't have to start out running the Boston Marathon; start with something small, something to build your confidence with and something you can someday accomplish.

When you're making a goal try setting a timeframe to accomplish the goal. Realize that some goals may take a lifetime and other goals may be accomplished in no time at all. I'm a firm believer that if no timeframe is set, your goal is nothing more than a dream. It just keeps going and going and going, and at some point will become an "I wish I would have." Ask yourself, how many I wish I would haves are hanging in your closet.

Don't get me wrong, every goal has multiple steps that need to be completed. I call these micro goals and it's these micro goals that must be accomplished to achieve the big one. To turn the aforementioned dream into a goal, it should sound something like "I'm going to run The Marine Corp Marathon in July." Simply changing the statement and adding a few words makes this a goal and now we work on the micro goals so we can achieve running the marathon.

Maybe you're thinking, "That's just a play on words, they both mean the same thing."

Do they?

I don't think so!

The reason I don't feel they mean the same is simple, the word will! I consider "will" a call to action word. Let's break this down a bit further.

Examples: I wish I could go on a cruise. I want to go on a cruise someday; I will go on a cruise.

Look at these examples: "*I wish I could go on a cruise*" vs. "I will go on a cruise." A few simple words can makes a difference mentally in regards to what someone will do with his or her goals as opposed to just wishing or thinking about them.

When you tell yourself "I will" or "I'm going to…" these words really have power and meaning. They can get you going on the right track to achieve any goal you set. Don't get me wrong, as I described above, there are micro goals you need to achieve to reach your overall goal. In the instance of going on the cruise the micro goals might be saving up money, getting off work, etc.

2 SET YOUR GOAL

Life goals come in all different shapes and sizes. It all starts when young boys and girls are asked what they want to be when they grow up.

From a young age, kids usually envision themselves as whoever the influential person in their life is at that time. If you catch a little boy on the baseball diamond, he may want to be the next big professional baseball player. If you ask that little girl playing dress up, she might reply, "I want to be the next pop star."

At this young age, children are impressionable by what's going on around them. The average child isn't thinking about what their goals in life are going to be. At this time, it is about having fun and being a kid.

If you are reading this, don't mistake this for you or your child. You want your child to be above average and to know what he or she wants to be; you will see it in his or her eyes. You will see that he or she wants that extra practice or just gets what it takes to make it big. You have to remember that he or she is still a kid and needs to be a kid. Encourage your child to work hard, harder than the other kids, but at the end of the day to go back to being a kid with his or her friends.

At this age— most kids don't even know they are setting small goals; "I'm going to score a touchdown at my next game," and at their next game, they run as hard as they can to try and score that touchdown, trying to accomplishing their goal. Even at a young age, as we teach, they are learning that even though they set goals, little things may be out of their control that could hold them back from actually achieving their goals.

As children mature, they start to understand the meaning and depth of setting their goals…they start to realize they need others' help and begin to rely on a parent, coach or someone they look up to. They understand they can't do it by themselves, once they realize this; they have set their foundation to success. Their personal goals will have much more meaning to them and so will learning to achieve each goal they set, whether or not they are successfully achieved.

Failure is part of success and will be a part of conquering your goal. It will be a long road to success and there will be times you fail on the way; as long as there is progress in learning how to accomplish specific goals and make the changes to do so, you will succeed. We call this "learning to adapt." Some may fail more than others while trying to achieve their goal; as it pertains to you, no matter how many times you fail, get up and keep going.

Don't be judged by your failures; be judged how you picked yourself up during those failures.

There are a lot of young people, who set goals at a young age, and for whatever reason, they fully understand the work that will go into achieving those goals, and there are also PARENTS who set goals for their children.

For this example, think of a dancer. This profession is extremely demanding, like other professions the hours that go into training are incredible, and the more involved the dancer is the more time is involved. If this is your goal, or your goal is similar, think of who is setting the goal. Do you really want to be a dancer, or do your parents want you to be a dancer? Do you want to be a dancer as a profession or is this just something to keep you busy? This is an example where it's important to question who setting the goal: a parent or a child? Are the hours dedicated to this passion out of the child's willpower, or is it the vicariousness of the parent? Unfortunately, in most cases, kids committed to these activities are living out their parents' dreams.

Far too often, I see parents living out their dreams through their children; it is truly a shame. There comes a time in life when parents need to let go of their childhood dreams, paint over memories and move on to the next phases of their lives.

A parent's primary role, is to be ultra supportive and objective about their child's activities; and to feel more proud of their child than of themselves at their own highest moment. The dream of becoming a great baseball player has passed, but pushing a child into something he or she may not want to do isn't right in any fashion. If it's the case that the child truly wants to be the next Broadway star, or even the next Olympian, you will see it in their eyes and hear it in their voice that they understand the commitment they need to take on to achieve that goal. Some parents get it, some don't; ultimately, you should let your child be great at what he or she is passionate about.

One moment during one of my coaching sessions with a parent stands out to me. The father really wanted his son to be a jock and play basketball but the child loved to read and work on computer programs. What was troubling when we first met was when the father told me the boy was ridiculed continuously by other boys because the son wasn't any good at basketball and the father was upset because the boy didn't stick up for himself while being made fun of. I asked the father, "why put him in the situation if he doesn't like basketball anyways?" Is he playing basketball because he wants to or because you want him to? The root of the problem was that the father was ashamed that his son wasn't athletic but, after a few coaching sessions the father began to see how great his son was at things other than sports. It made all the difference and actually made the father and son closer because the son was able to teach the father everything he loved to do.

Personally, I remember growing up and wanting to be the next Thurman Munson; he was the New York Yankees catcher in the 1970's. Oh, and I wanted to be a fireman and a truck driver; but wait, I wanted to be the next Walter Payton, the famous running back for the Chicago Bears. I was no different from any other child fantasizing about being someone I idolized. Like other kids, I thought it looked so simple to be that person(s) I looked up to. Not to mention, I had parents that patted my head and said, "You can be anything you want to be." I have to admit my parents were my biggest supporters of some of my crazier idea and goals in life.

I wanted to be all those things and it wasn't until I was older that I started to pinpoint what it was I wanted to focus on. My dreams weren't any different than anyone else's growing up; my dreams were bigger than life! Even today, as I sit on the bleachers of life and watch my own kids, I remember all the times my parents ran me to this practice and that practice to make me better. That's what it is about… making your kids, or yourself, better at what you are doing. Obviously, the Yankees weren't going to draft me at twelve years old, and I certainly wouldn't be allowed to be a truck driver at that age. Therefore, it's pretty easy to see the difference between goals and merely chasing dreams and trying to bank on wishes.

But, it's important to note that there are always exceptions to this rule. Maybe it's that incredible voice you hear singing in the choir and you just know that person will be the next star. Maybe it is that little league catcher that just stands out above everyone, and you know he will make it to the Big Leagues someday.

It's funny, maybe even ironic, when you hear a third party person being interviewed about that one great athlete and they recall, "I remember watching her tumble in gymnastics and I just knew she was going to make it to the Olympics." Often times, it only takes that one person to see in another's eyes that he or she has what it takes to achieve something special. It takes a special child, or person for that fact, to be able to achieve such greatness at such a young age. While some kids are out playing with friends, it's the inspired kid's prerogative to be in the gym, on the stage or in the library reading. Those traits of hard work are what set the future great ones apart from the others.

It's called DEDICATION!

Something in the brain clicks and the individual understands all the hard work that it is going to take to achieve what he or she has set out to do. It is okay to dream about becoming something better or making it to the next level. It keeps our minds and bodies fresh; don't EVER allow anyone to crush your dreams! You never know when that dream is going to become a goal and when that goal will become success. There will be doubters; rise above them and keep going.

3 CHANGING GOALS

Your goals change throughout your life. You might start out wanting to be a fireman as a child and then decide you'd prefer to be a school teacher as you get older. You have to understand that goals change. Always, carefully, take the next steps toward your goal. Look deep into your heart and ask yourself if this is what you really want to do, and whether or not you are settling.

Don't ever settle on a goal. If you want to be the next great professional athlete, then do it. Only you hold the key to make that happen. Sure, you will have people around you that are there to help, and people around to watch you fail. Failing is always a part of success; getting knocked down on your way to the top or being knocked down while at the top… either way, failing keeps you on your toes. You never want to look back and say I wish I would have. Always say "I remember when." Your best asset to yourself and to others is to use your successes to help others achieve theirs.

There will be times when life throws you a curveball, and sometimes you will hit it out of the ballpark; sometimes life will get the best of you. Those are the times when you should look at your goal and make a few adjustments; learn to adapt to each scenario. Don't ever let anyone tell you that you are ridiculous in wanting to set any goal you want. I would never sit here and say all your goals you set are going to be achieved or loved by people in your life that care for you. People are very judgmental and throughout your life as you set goals you will always have your few that—no matter what—will try and put you down for what you want to do. Generally, it's jealousy that causes others to want to see you fail. They are jealous because you are taking steps toward your goal, while leaving them behind to sit and ponder their dreams. There are factors that are sometimes out of your control that might hinder you from what you have set out to achieve. You will learn to adapt and you might even have to put certain goals on the shelf until later, but never ever give up.

You should always try and circle yourself with great and supportive people. No one has ever conquered one of their goals all by themselves. Behind every great athlete are great coaches, parents and teammates. Likewise, behind every great astronaut are teachers and mentors that helped that special person achieve his or her ultimate goal. It's important to never forget that. Look to others for inspiration and for the fuel to keep going. It's okay to ask for help, advice or a pep talk. Asking for help does not betray weakness, it shows you don't know everything and want to learn; learning is part of the process of succeeding.

Can you remember one of your first goals? Was it making

the all-star team, the junior varsity or the varsity team? Was it wanting to go to college to play the sport you loved, or trying out at the local professional sports combine hoping to make it to the bigs? If you get to the show (the show is a term for making it to the majors), then what? Do you finish your education, go to grad school and take the next step to your next big goal? All of these are all legitimate goals you might set for yourself.

Every step of the way will get harder and harder. The numbers get tighter and tighter on how many make it to each level. I've spoken to so many athletes and future business owners that gave up even before getting started. They listened to everyone around them telling them how hard it was to make it in business or a given sport and how many people don't make it, and left it at that. They didn't push the naysayer to tell them, "if you really believe in yourself and work hard, you just might make yourself one of those few that make it."

Don't get me wrong, the numbers demonstrate the amount of people who don't make it and fail the first time. The first time, but what about the second time or third? They don't know how hard you work and how deeply your desire to be successful; they don't realize that you aren't looking for the easy road.

But is that you? You are reading this book because you want that edge, the motivation to keep going. When things get tough, you have to reach deep inside yourself and keep pushing toward your goal. It's hard to hear the words "Don't Give Up" from others. You think to yourself, "They don't understand what it takes to get through this practice in 100 degree heat in full pads," or what is like to feel like your lungs are going to burn out of your chest while running that marathon. They don't understand what it might be like to work 18 hour days running a business while knowing it might fail.

Instead of thinking, "the others don't have a clue," because, unless they are walking in your shoes, you are right they don't know what you are going through, they are giving you the almighty, "I really don't care but keep your chin up," rah rah rah speech. What you need to do is channel that energy to help you. Though they may not be you nor understand what you are going through, they are the people you want around you to motivate you to keep going. They don't have to understand the pain and suffering you are experiencing. They only need to support you. So take that "rah rah rah" and energize yourself. Ask any great athlete, or business owner; it's the support that kept and keeps them going, before during and after making it to the top.

4 IS YOUR GOAL REALISTIC?

This, by far, will be one of the hardest things to talk about: being realistic with your goals. Like most, I've grown up listening to people constantly telling me "you can't do this," or "you can't do that; just be like so and so." It was the hardest thing to hear. The constant beat down, by others will wear on you, but, be strong. Remember it's easier to put someone down than it is to support them. Keep that in the back of your mind through your ups and downs.

I remember sitting in the guidance counselor's office and talking about college and baseball and football scholarships and being told by the counselor, I would be nothing more than a ditch digger. I was told that college wasn't for me and that I should focus on factory or construction jobs, I looked at that guidance counselor and said, "No, I'm going to college." Before leaving his office I looked him in the eyes across his desk and said with a strong, stern, 17-year-old voice: "If that is all I will be, I'll be the best ditch digger there is."

Even though I went to college, I've always taken offense when people talk down about construction workers, truck drivers or factory workers. "I would be proud to be a ditch digger because they built this school we are sitting in and the roads we drive on to get us to school," I continued. He just looked at me as I walked out the door. (I had a passion for the construction trade through family members that were in the trade).

As you are setting your goals, be proud of whatever you become and do it 100%. To this day, when telling that story to groups, I look at peoples expressions and it's clear that so many have heard similar statements. That is when being motivated and believing in yourself is so important. Don't allow someone behind a desk to steal your dreams. Don't allow your drive to succeed to be diminished because that person doesn't see in you what you see in yourself. Look that person in the eye and nicely say, "sir or ma'am, I understand the uphill battle that is in front of me to accomplish my goal and achieve success, but I also understand the hard work I need to put in to make my goal become a reality. I'm sorry you don't believe in me, but I believe in me!"

I spoke in the last section about living your dreams and trying to make your dreams into reality, I truly believe that. I believe if you set out to achieve a specific goal you can do it.

I also believe that you have to be realist.

You are probably tilting your head right now because I just

spoke about not giving up and said that you can accomplish anything. You can! But now I say you need to be a realist when setting your goals.

Being a realist isn't contradictory to being able to achieve anything you set your mind to. Instead, it's about understanding the fight it will take to achieve your goal. The road blocks will be endless and you have to be mentally prepared for them at any age.

I often think while watching kids at an event, whether at a pee-wee football game or on the stage, that I can pick out the ones that are or could really be someone special. Their voices are just that much better or their moves on the football field just flow better than any other players. I wonder if they know they are special.

Every parent thinks their child is special and in some cases may over look their actual ability...both good and bad. I don't think there is any parent out there that wants their child to go out and not succeed in a game or competition. Some parents will be a little more aggressive in how a child is doing and some will just be okay with whatever performance is given and might congratulate them for just doing it. A point can be made for both types. One can say the outcome doesn't matter and cheer their child on while another parent can hold that perspective that win or lose the child needs to be told what he or she did wrong and needs to work on. The important question is, does the child actually realize that he or she has a gift to be great, or not?

In most cases at this stage in a child's life, it is more about having fun, running around and being with friends; it's the parents doing the pushing. I spoke about wanting to be the next Walter Payton while running with the football behind the elementary school on a Sunday morning in the fall. Did I really think I would be the next great running back? Sure I did. I wore the same game jersey and had my cleats and I made moves like him, in my eyes I was Walter Payton. But at twelve I was just that kid playing football in the back yard with his friends.

You are asking yourself how am I to know at such a young age if I want to be the next super star. It's simple... You will just know. People around you will see something in you that you may not see in yourself. Maybe you run faster than the other kids. Maybe you have this ability to see the ball better in your given sport. You just might have this incredible personality that just yells, "super star." As a singer maybe it's a great voice that makes you stand out. My point is that there is something that sets you apart from everyone else.

You are probably even more confused now. I'm about to explain why, I'm illustrating a pattern throughout the book, of being a realist; I think it's most important to be a realist when making your goals. You probably have people thinking they are helping you with what they think would be a great goal for you, maybe it's an over-bearing parent that really wants you to make it at what he or she wants you to become, maybe it's a parent who is trying to live his or her life through you and that's why you're being pushed toward a certain goal. You work tirelessly on the courts, diamonds, and/or the stage, with coach after coach and for what? For you or for your parents and their dreams? You have to ask yourself is this for you or for them? Look deep within yourself and be honest with yourself and those pushing you at something you just aren't interested in.

I've taken this stance with my own children or while speaking to people about motivating their kids. Kids are kids; you won't change that. Parents and kids both need to understand that they need kid time. It's okay to push kids just like you push adults. But remember, as adults we can say with comfort, "I need a break" kids on the other hand will need our guidance in setting them free of training and letting them return to the fun things in life. As a parent you need to realize when they mentally just can't take anymore. Kids will check out mentally long before you or the coach will. Learn when that happens, and you will be successful both as a parent and coach and you will have a much more driven child because you'll know they checked out mentally and you will be able to say that's the end of practice.

I would rather get the best half hour or hour of practice then drag something on for hours and hours and achieve nothing. Yes, nothing is what you will get out of them; after you lose them mentally, not only do you as a coach get frustrated because of the mistakes or lack of enthusiasm but the kids will actually go backwards with their training and it won't take long to lose them all together. That's why it's so important to get the most out of you or your child when you have his or her attention. You can't change kids being kids.

Too often, you hear of adults that took a different path from the one their parents had set up for them. During these conversations you hear these young grownups talk about not having a childhood growing up, because their parents always had them training. You need to understand that these kids will eventually grow up, their bodies will change, goals will change and lives will change. But, the adults that say these things weren't kids that set their own goals, their parents set them for them. They didn't want to play the sport anymore and were afraid to disappoint their parents or coaches so they just kept playing. I, personally, think this is wrong on so many levels.

Ask your kids, "do you want to play this or do that?" Let them tell you "NO, "and if they do, ask what they want to do.

I would rather a child give a 100% in something they love than give 5% in something they hate.

Remember, in some cases if it's a team sport, other kids may be giving 100% because they want to be there and if your child isn't giving his or her fare share of effort that can make it tough on so many levels.

It's frustrating to hear how some parents and children are so narrow-minded about being realists. I always talk about taking the blinders off and seeing the big picture. Learn to adapt to change and embrace it.

I remember this one time I was speaking to a father about his son and how he wanted him to be the next great quarterback. Let me say that the kid had great potential. He possessed a good arm and was able to really understand his defense's reads. This child was ten and playing pee-wee football. The father spoke of Division 1 football scholarships and how they train all summer and how his child was going to be the next great quarterback.

I remember talking with the child/quarterback and asking him what he thought? I asked him alone and with his dad. When with his dad he was just as pumped and spoke of being the next big thing in the quarterback world, but when alone it was refreshing to hear him talk about why he wouldn't make it as a Division 1 player. The child was being a realist but the dad wasn't seeing past his blinders. The child realized he probably wasn't going to be tall enough to make it at that level of play. But also, he just wasn't sure he even wanted it. He wanted to focus on his education and realized there was an extremely high probability that he wouldn't make the pro's so he wanted to play the game for fun and not because he felt he had to.

Don't get me wrong, there are kids out there that understand they have all the tools to be great at that level of play and nothing will stand in their way to get there, their goals are different, the realization that they might make it is real and they truly feel their goal is attainable.

Being a life coach and mentor to this family was difficult but I had to speak up; I spoke with the father about looking at the big picture. The big picture is about being a realist; the father stands 5'9 and the mother 5'3. The family height history is about the same on both sides. I explained to my friend that he had no idea what his child's height would end up being. Sure, the doctors can chart an approximate height but he'd never know the final outcome until his son was done growing. I told the father there was always the possibility his son would make it and that it would take a lot of work but that, even with enough hard work, there was the possibility he might not make it to the level he wanted or his child wanted. I told him his son should have a back-up goal just in case and to always keep an open mind to change.

This goes for all parents, it's extremely important that, as parents, we keep an open mind about change. We need to be supportive no matter what. We should be mentors throughout the process.

My job as a motivational coach is to make people see the whole field (no pun intended). What is seeing the whole field? It's looking at the big picture…trying to visualize the end product of what the goal is, and then working backwards in researching what and who, with similar stats as your child has already achieved the same goal. Breaking down your goal this way allows you to see who has already achieved something similar and what they went through to get there. Don't reinvent the wheel unless it needs to be reinvented.

Learning to adapt is the most important lesson you need to learn in accomplishing your goal. It's the first step in realizing if you love it enough to make it your career or if it should it just be for fun. Do you have all the tools you need to make it? At twelve, most kids have no idea if they have what it takes to make it. It's others who will see a glimmer of something that a child does that just amazes them and those people will push him or her to the next level…

A child isn't fully grown in mind or body to fully understand if he or she will have what it takes. As children grow more mature, they will feel it. They will see other kids around the sport or activity they are in and realize if they have what it takes or not. They will seek that extra help to make themselves better. They will watch film on their techniques. They will work harder than anyone else on their performance; they will see that the goal will become clearer in their minds.

5 ADAPT!

Too many times, I've seen kids give up their goals because they didn't get the starting quarterback position, they weren't starting forward on the soccer team or they weren't the lead in the play. This is where you have to adapt. Maybe you are too short, not fast enough or maybe your hands are too small, maybe you just can't sing; it might be out of your hands and maybe a coach doesn't or teacher just doesn't see you in that starting role; regardless of the reason, don't give up...adapt and conquer.

For whatever reason, don't give up the goal of being a star. Find that position or even that sport that you stand out in. Maybe it isn't the lead that makes you shine. Maybe you are a supporting part of the play or team that really shows your true colors. It is about learning how to adapt to a situation while still making that situation come out in your favor.

I remember the first time I saw the movie "Rudy." Rudy had a dream of going to Notre Dame and playing football but there was obstacle after obstacle that he had to overcome. Whether it was his size, lack of support from his family or bad grades...whatever the obstacle was he overcame it. His dream of playing football for Notre Dame became a goal and he was going to do anything to achieve that goal. Those obstacles were micro goals and he conquered each micro goal along the way to achieve the main goal.

The movie is inspirational in many ways and sad in others. People take from it what they want to get out of it. Personally, it taught me to never give up on any goal or dream. In the movie, Rudy was trying to prove so many people wrong in his town and family, that when he didn't achieve his goal at first he was only ridiculed more. In turn he used that ridicule to push himself further and ultimately achieved his goal. It's a great motivating tool I use it to this day when I need to refocus my energy to the goal I have set for myself. Always remember that it's easier for people to ridicule or be jealous of someone than to provide support.

6 WORKING TOWARD YOUR GOAL

In the last few sections I spoke of the ups and downs of goals and dreams and the people behind you helping you achieve what you are setting out to accomplish along with the naysayers.

This section is about helping you work toward your goal. The famous phrase coaches and parents use is "work hard." I see that as common sense. Of course you have to work hard. Let's take that phrase and build on it. Let's use that phrase as our foundation to success.

Now, we have to build on top of our foundation.

First, ask yourself what you think it takes to accomplish your goal. We have established that hard work is essential. But, "hard work" is such a broad statement. It doesn't pin point one specific area that will help you achieve anything. You are probably scratching your head now.

Let's use the example of golf. Your coach or parents

constantly say "you have to work hard." That doesn't really help, does it? You need specifics, what is it you need to work hard on? Is that work hard at your chipping or maybe putting? Then you hear the brilliant phrase "You have to work harder." Harder at what again you ask? Most times you have to realize if someone isn't fully educated regarding your sport it's easier to make a comment like that, take it with a grain of salt and use it to keep you going, pushing you toward your goal.

Let's talk about repetitions and working hard during those repetitions; you need to get reps in to become better. You don't get better by doing an exercise once. You get better by doing it 100 times. But you need to make sure you are doing the rep right. It doesn't help if you are doing the movement wrong, right? Of course it doesn't. So before you go out and start doing rep after rep, make sure your technique is right: quality over quantity.

Let's break it down step by step, remembering what we already said in earlier chapters about learning to adapt. Another important aspect of becoming great to an athlete or performer is to take off the blinders and have thick skin. These are two important things to learn if you want to be the next great thing. What is thick skin? It is a metaphor for being able to take criticism. When you stand out from the others on your team or other performers, you are going to have times throughout your life that others will put you down or criticize how you do things. These are the times you will need thick skin. You will have to learn how to deal with this criticism and learn how to not let it bother you. I know it will be easier said than done but trust me, you are strong enough to deal with this and move past it to keep on track and conquer your goals. In life you will always have someone that doesn't like you, whether it's a coworker, maybe a neighbor or a teacher; someone out there will always not like you. Shrug your shoulders at it and move on.

Take off the blinders, look around and watch; watch and take everything in, "the good the bad and the ugly." Watch what others do great on the team. Watch the ones that don't do so great and watch the ones who work so hard and will never get any better but they keep trying. Why? Any performer, whether athletic or not needs to see what's around them. You can build yourself off the talent around you. If you have someone that I described above that will just never get better but has so much heart, feed off that individual; feed off his or her heart and desire wanting to get better. This person can help you to never settle; always try to better yourself.

When it comes to competition—whether fighting for a starting position, the lead role or trying to move up the corporate ladder—it's important to know the good the bad and the ugly. It doesn't matter if you are twelve or forty; I'm a firm believer in knowing all aspects of your position and others' positions while watching your opponents and their techniques.

You should be a master at your position/job. You should want to know everything there is to know. But, it doesn't stop there; a great player will know what the others around him are doing. If it's football, the running back will know what the lineman are doing on any given play. If it's an actress, she will know not only her lines but others so she can understand the scene. If it's the CEO, he should know not only the financials of the company but how the company works from top to bottom. Never just settle for knowing what you have to do, look around and know everything that is going on: the good, the bad and the ugly.

The good

I use this term, THE GOOD, because no matter what time in your life you are in, you have to look at the good in yourself and others around you. That's not just how good someone is in a performance but also as a person. In order for you to succeed, you need to circle yourself with good people, people who believe in themselves and also believe in you.

You have learned by now that you have to get to know your opposing team, opponent or competing company. Look at what makes them good. Maybe it's how they are built. Maybe it's an eye for the ball. Maybe it's their work ethic as you watch them train. Maybe it's how they eat. Maybe it's their attitude as a whole that sets them apart. There are so many things that could make up a great person or team that I could go on and on about them. In order to keep growing yourself, never assume you are done learning and definitely don't think you know everything. Keep an open mind and look at others who have succeeded. Look at the path they took to get them there and see what you can learn from them to conquer your goal. The people who believe in you are here to help you succeed, to help you reach your goal.

This is where learning to adapt is so important. Don't ever and I mean ever be anyone other than YOU! I gave the examples of wanting to be Thurman Munson and Walter Payton; I didn't actually want to be them specifically. I wanted to be great at my position like them.

It's not the cleats that make the runner great; it's the runner in those cleats.

It's so important to learn to be the best you can be. Be the athlete and person that best fits you.

The Bad

Every group, team or sport has them and to accomplish your goal you need to be able to deal with the bad and ugly of the team and sport. In trying to accomplish your goal you need to be able to channel the issues that will stand in front of you. Whether you're part of a team sport or a sport that is just about you, you will experience all kinds of characters that can stand in your way of reaching your potential as a great athlete, performer or career person. You have to learn to take the bad and ugly of others on your team and channel their energy to your goal. Not everyone will have the same goals as you and you need to realize that and be able to deal with Barb or Billy not caring if the performance went off without a hitch, if you won or lost the game or if the company is profitable or not.

This is about being a team player. It's good to have a competitive spirit but don't let that competitive spirit spill over into being a sore loser or an arrogant winner. If the boss picks your presentation over someone else's, congratulate them for doing a good job; remember they worked hard on the project also. There is always a winner and loser and someday you maybe on the losing end and you wouldn't want to be treated any less than how you will treat someone.

Now, let's be a realist and realize this is the real world and you just might find yourself on the other end of someone that doesn't take winning or losing very well and is just plan rude. Remember you have thick skin; don't let it bother you! Learning from your competitors will only make you a better.

Personally, I can remember watching other catchers growing up both professionally and my age, studying their moves and seeing what they did wrong. Maybe it was their stance on different pitches or how they called the game for the pitcher, maybe it was their release throwing the ball to second; I looked at everything, the good, the bad and the ugly. I made sure I worked toward not making the same mistakes and focused on things to make me better.

You need to remember that foundation you are building to help you conquer your goal; the building blocks, your "teammates" may not always be as strong as you like and it's your job to strengthen those blocks. Learn to teach and work for the common goal of becoming better not only as a single player but as a team… sounds a lot like we are building a LEADER. A good leader is like the team cheerleader, you are the motivator of the team, when down you know how to pick them up. Please always remember, people generally don't fail on purpose; the actor doesn't purposely flub his or her lines, the outfielder doesn't purposely drop the ball. The people who made the mistake feel bad enough, they don't need others to come down on them…pick them up; the mistake is in the past and can't be changed so keep moving forward toward the goal.

The single most important thing to remember is to stay positive. Someone will make a mistake and you will need to step up as the leader and motivator to keep their spirits up. You know they feel horrible for making the mistake; but, you still need them as your building block so build them up, don't break them down. If you break them down your foundation only weakens.

The Ugly

Working with the ugly is and will be a task most will just walk away from and not deal with. These are the athletes or performers who may never get it or don't even want to be there, but have parents that are living through them and making them participate in something they just aren't interested in. You might have a coworker that feels stuck in their job and just puts in as much effort needed to keep his or her job; these people do exist and do have the ability to alter your goals. In any case you need to tackle (not literally) these areas of weakness in others head on if you want to make it to the top. Maybe you can make Mary or Bob see something in their job they might like that gives them a new sense of passion for what they do. Not only will this be important for the team, but also for you as a person. Being a team player will pump a feeling through your veins like no other.

The feeling you will experience when you help that one person is so incredible; it will catapult you to another level of success and one step closer to achieving your goal. Take the ugly and work with them. It will not only help with your personal achievement but will help your own skill level as it teaches you at the same time as them. It's teaching you the same techniques and remember, I said earlier repetition is the name of the game; do it over and over and become great at it. You will find yourself frustrated at times, but take those frustrating moments and build off them; teach yourself how to keep your cool under pressure. Other coaches, parents or coworkers will see the help you are giving to the ones that need it and it will set you apart from the ones who don't have the leadership qualities you do. You need to acknowledge that in some cases, no matter how hard you work to help someone, they may just never get it…keep looking at your techniques and keep trying. Remember, you need to conquer your goal and in some cases it's not as easy as drafting in the right help; you have to learn to work with what is around you and keep building them up to greatness!

Being a leader is the hardest thing for most to accept. I'm a believer that leaders are born and not made. You are either a leader or you aren't. Taking charge of your goal starts with being a leader. Remember, leaders always need help in reaching their goals also; a good leader is a good motivator and can motivate others to not only accomplish his or her goal, but the goals of others.

7 PHYSICAL PREPARATION

A machine is *a tool consisting of one or more parts that is constructed to achieve a particular goal.* Think of your body as a machine that is built to a specific specification to run at full power and to achieve the outputs that its owner is expecting.

You have to build your body to a specification that is best used in the achievement of the goal set forth by you, its owner. Whatever activity you are involved in will have a desired body type or specific physical traits that would be most efficient in achieving your goal. I'm a firm believer that you need to build your body in a way that is best suited for you. You are born with certain traits and no matter how much lifting, dieting and lessons you undertake, you were given certain traits that just can't be changed. Here is where you need to adapt, and be a realist.

Once you have adapted your goal that best fits your abilities, it's time to build your physique. This isn't just for sports. Even a singer needs to be in shape for the rigors of being on stage for hours, professions have certain physical criteria's that need to be met, it's so important you follow a workout that best fits you. You are you; you aren't Derek Jeter or Brittney Spears, but their workouts are tailored to their sport and body and you will need to do the same. What works for them may not work for you. Your sport and/or career will dictate the type of workout you will need to do for the most part. Some careers may not need a specific body type but overall I'm not promoting you try to be Barbie and Ken, I'm promoting good health, even if it's just for the sake of your loved ones.

If you pick up any weight training magazine you will see your typical reps and sets that are widely used for publication. Don't think if you follow that specific work out and diet that you will look like the person in the magazine. Sure you might get a little bigger or you might even tighten up but the overall outcome will be basic. It kills me how these youth programs only have basic workouts for sports. Let's use football as an example; some coaches have running backs lifting the same as lineman. These are two totally different positions and each workout needs tailored for that specific position and body type. You may be that running back reading this and nodding your head. Don't get me wrong any work out is better than not working out at all. If you are in a position that won't allow you a specific workout tailored to you, then work hard at what you are given and make the best of it.

This phase isn't going to be all peaches and cream. This phase is going to test you. You are the one with the goal, you are going to have to put in some extra hours working on specific movements and exercises for your position or sport. It doesn't matter if this is sports-related or career-related; you want to be the best you can. Whether it's at your tennis game or putting in the hours on rotations, be the best you can be!

What is universal is keeping motivated; even seasoned athletes need that pick-me-up, it could be a song or quote to keep them or you going. I spoke earlier about losing one's attention after a certain amount of time, well that goes for adults also. Make meetings short and to the point, don't let them drag on and on, if you do, you will only lose the attention of the people you need to help you accomplish your goals. When you are at your lowest is when keeping yourself motivated will be the hardest. For me, it's when things are going great that I have a tough time staying motivated. When things get tough, I know I have to pull up my boot straps, dig in and work hard. But, if I've reached my goal and need to maintain that goal, that is when sometimes I lose focus and slide backwards. Don't allow that to happen to you. Keep strong and focused. Realize that just because you made it to your goal, you still have to maintain it. What has helped me is good eating habits; a healthy body needs healthy eating. Eating healthy is one of the key aspects of conquering your goal.

Why, you may ask?

I don't know of many successful athletes or others that have been champions or overly successful in their field, on the "oversize me" or "biggie meal plan." Sumo wrestlers don't count and don't get me wrong there are overweight people who hold very successful positions in life and there are positions in life and sports that may need you to carry a few extra pounds. But, there are risk factors in doing so, and let's be honest, we live in a society that stereotypes EVERYONE! You may need to really check to see how thick your skin is, because anything outside of what society considers the norm is usually made fun of or criticized. I personally think it's B.S. but everyone has an opinion.

I also don't believe in totally taking away your comfort food, the "makes me feel good food." You have to learn as an athlete training or any training for that matter, that everything is okay in moderation. You have to realize that your body burns far more energy than the average person. Just like working out, eating healthy will be hard work and mentally challenging.

Let me be brutally honest with you; unless you are mentally ready to change your lifestyle and make that leap to a healthy one, don't waste your time or anyone else's. Fooling yourself into thinking you are ready because Billy or Bobby Sue is eating salads and you want to do what they are doing because you think they are healthy can and will only send you on a whirlwind path of disaster. If you don't see changes in your lifestyle from eating right or even through exercise right away, it could cause you to fall further behind with your goals. It's all mental!

Think about it; as your buddies or girlfriends are sitting at your favorite fast food joint, pounding down the double whatever with a large fry and a milkshake while you are working on a chicken salad with a bottle of water, be prepared to hear their ridicule. Whether you want to call it peer pressure or a different name, don't allow it to beat you. Your friends or coworkers will always question why you are on a diet. But, DO NOT call it a diet, use the phrase "eating healthy." You aren't dieting; you are making a conscious decision to fill your body with the right foods to get you to the finish line. You need the right calories and proteins at the right times to feed the machine. It doesn't matter if you are the starting quarterback, the pop star on tour or the office secretary, eating right is essential to having a great day.

Remember the earlier reference to the machine. If you don't change the oil in the car, what happens? The machine breaks down. Your body is no different. Feed the machine the wrong foods long enough and it will break down. It's okay to take that cheat day and enjoy a special meal, whatever your special meal might be. It helps, shake up your metabolism anyways and I know from my personal experiences it just tastes good every once in a while. Don't get me wrong, when you eat healthy but you are craving something bad and you go for that comfort food, there are consequences and I would keep myself close to a bathroom, because your body will react accordingly.

Just like working out, you need to find what eating habit best fits your sport and lifestyle.

A swimmer's eating habits are far different than a tennis player's; an offensive lineman's calorie intake will be different than a quarterback's. A movie actor's eating habits for a role may be different than a famous singer's. Be sure to tailor your nutritional needs according to what you need. Magazines are notorious in printing the newest fad in eating to gain or lose pounds. Now obviously, at the bottom of each ad is the fine print that says it only helps a certain percentage of people who exercise correctly…blah blah blah. In layman's terms, you need to work out and eat right for anything to work.

There isn't a magical pill out there (well there is, but under a doctor's prescription) or a magical eating regimen that will help the masses. It's important to find out what is the best for you. I know I said that once before but drill that sentence in your memory. It has to be right for you.

I remember at one time when I was lifting and Dorian Yates was Mr. Olympia. I tried his workout and eating habits and did this religiously. Guess what, they didn't do a thing for me. Our bodies were different types, our metabolisms were different and I wasn't taking the supplements he was. But, you would have sworn by reading the magazine that if you followed Dorian's workouts and eating habits you could be just like him. It was all about selling magazines. Feed off what others want to achieve and put words in big red text and it can make you feel like you can do it. It's great marketing but not reality. Now, I didn't think I was going to be the next Mr. Olympia, but I was naïve and thought I would have achieved what I was looking for. I am here to say, NO!

I didn't give up!

I did more reading and even after not gaining anything from my workouts like Dorian, I figured I would do the workouts for six weeks to see if I would get any improvement. That's a good time frame to follow when trying to figure out if something's going to work for you.

It's a perfect time for your body to adjust to something new and enough time to experience minute losses or gains you might be looking for. If like me, you don't get the results you desire, don't give up and get discouraged. Don't go jumping on the triple-size-me burger bender or the next quick fad. Keep your course and shoot for the next training cycle of eating habits and/or workouts and see how they might work. Please remember this, you just worked out for six weeks, you might not have seen the gains or losses you were expecting, but you just worked out for six weeks; that sure is better than doing nothing. All isn't lost, it's a micro goal. You just completed a small goal toward your overall goal, you learned how to adapt. See how this is all fitting into your life?

Don't be afraid to ask for help. People so often are afraid to ask for the simple things in life from the people that would love to help. Talk to a local trainer or someone in that specific area of expertise and pick the brain of the knowledge you seek to help you achieve your goal. People love to talk about things they are passionate about, suck their brain dry of as much knowledge as you can. It doesn't matter if it's a professor in the career field you want to go in or someone with more knowledge than you might have. You always have room to learn and get better.

I can't stress enough, to get to the top of that mountain and claim your goal; your eating habits and staying healthy are some of the most important things you will need to accomplish in your search to be the best you can be.

Not only will your body thank you for it, your mind will rejoice also.

Strong body, Strong mind!

8 MENTAL PREPARATION

Everyone at some point has heard the term "strong mind, strong body." Well that is true! If you aren't mentally prepared to try and accomplish your goal than it's time to get you prepared.

This concept will be one of the easiest for me to explain but one of the hardest for you to achieve.

It's often said that the strong survive and the weak die. I always wondered when I heard that saying, what it meant. Does it refer to physical strength? So the people next to me that can lift a house will survive before I do?

No!

It wasn't until I was in the Air Force that I figured it out. The phrase is talking about the strong willed. In the military they were trying to teach us that no matter what the circumstances you are facing may be you need to keep your cool and accomplish the mission. It wouldn't matter

46

how strong your body was, it was how strong your mind was able to deal with everything that was going on around you. It might be something as simple as 50-below temperatures or gun fire buzzing by your head, as you crawl through mud and barbwire. Whatever the situation is, it's your mind that needs to be strong and again that is easier said than done.

Stress, stress, stress!!!

Stress can play a major factor (in my opinion) in holding you back from achieving your ultimate goals. You have to minimize your stress the best you can. Remember, earlier in the book I talked about being a realist. Well this is one of those times. Stress is all around us. It's being caught in traffic, a friend's drama at school, it's the midterm you have coming up, it's the big date Saturday night, it's the game on Friday, a co-worker being a real pain in the derriere, and gas prices. It's all around you! I could keep going and going but that might stress you out. You have to learn how to channel that stress into positive energy.

You have to learn to let stress roll off your shoulders. By this point, you have thickened your skin and now it's time to utilize that new trait. That's easier said than done. But let's break it down, getting caught in traffic, NOT stressful. It's more of a pain in the butt. Rising gas prices, NOT stressful, it's upsetting and all you can do is change your driving habits, ultimately it is just a pain, not stressful. You have to pinpoint actual stressful situations compared to situations that are just annoying and usually out of your control. These two examples are out of your overall control, you don't control the fuel market and you certainly don't control the 405, but you can control how you deal with these stressors. You can always drive the speed limit, get a smaller car and take a different route so ultimately you can control your stress to a certain extent.

Stressful would be losing your job or a critically ill family member. Situations like these are stressful and will take every bit of mental control you have to deal with. In tough scenarios like these, you may have to adapt your goal; it may get put on hold or changed all together. The great thing about adapting goals is that you get to reinvent yourself! Life-changing situations can actually be life-changing for everyone around you and sometimes can be used as wake-up calls to propel you forward.

Mentally learning to adapt your goals to life will make you a better athlete, employee and person. Every day people just give up on their goals because a life-changing event happens. When talking with athletes, I like to use an issue like a knee injury. In a lot of cases an ACL tear is the end-all to anyone's career. There are exceptions, and usually there are many factors that make up those exceptions. If you have an injury that is catastrophic, your mental toughness will come into play during your rehab. Mentally preparing yourself for an injury is impossible. At the moment that injury happens and you are laying there in pain and then sitting in the doctor's office listening to the news that you will never play your sport again, never finish the career you love, may never sing again or act again is the most gut-wrenching experience. There is no doubt your mind will want to fail you at first. You will want to give up. You will be mad at the world and want to crawl under the nearest rock.

WHY???

Obviously, certain injuries can end one's career. But ADAPT, remember: be strong mentally you are a great. Pull up your boot straps, shake your head and get back at it. You may have to reinvent yourself. It may be in a totally different arena or often times in a different sport or position all together; it might be an entirely different career. If you hurt your back and you are a fireman and you can't lift or run or do what it takes to do that career anymore, it's time to adapt, to change, to reinvent yourself; if you conquered your goal of being a fireman at some point in your life, it's time to conquer your next goal you set for yourself.

In some cases life spans in some careers are short anyways and a lot of sports life spans are even shorter, so learning to adapt and enjoying other sports or activities will be a key to your success overall.

The old saying "don't put all your eggs in one basket," is true.

It's important to have other interests, something to fall back on should you need to adapt to change quickly. You can evolve in other areas of your expertise like education, personalized instruction, etc. Don't use the injury as an excuse to let everything go; use it as a tool to help others…think of you as an asset. I'll keep using sports as an example. Often times, when players get injured they stay on as coaches. Often times, companies use injured employees from home if they can't make it into the office. Don't feel as if you can't keep going, because you can, you just might need to think outside of the box and adapt.

Using your mind to help heal your body is extremely important obviously, but, using your mind to push you to the next level is equally important. I'm sure you have heard of a runner's high? It's that time when your body hits that point and you feel like you can't go any further and then "BOOM" it's like your mind hits a switch that tells every muscle in your body to keep going; your mind is telling your muscles "it's okay, we got this." Your mind is such an amazing machine; utilize it to your fullest potential.

9 GAME DAY

Game day... The Mind... The Body... YOUR GOAL...

Is your mind ready? Didn't we just talk about your mind in the last section? We did. We talked about how strong of an asset it is and how it will help you accomplish your goals.

How does that work on game day? Game day can mean different things to different people. It isn't always sports-related. It might be that big presentation or that big lunch meeting to close a deal. It could be that big tour you are starting with your band. Game day means something different to every person.

Let's break it down.

Whether you are ten or forty; a professional or weekend warrior athlete; a seasoned entertainer or first-timer on the stage, having a clear head on game day is the foundation of success. The butterflies you feel in your belly and having to run to the bathroom to throw up is normal. This feeling will subside as you become more comfortable in your craft but there will be instances those butterflies will return from time to time.

Staying focused is key to your success When you are up against a 4mph cross wind, the cup is tucked in the far back of the green and the sand trap sits feet away, focus on that task at hand. To clear your mind and focus, paint your mind with your favorite color, use that imaginary paint to cover up any nervousness you might feel or anything that might keep you from being able to focus, keep the stresses behind closed doors.

Tell yourself you are going to do the best you can and do it. No matter what the outcome there will be times you gave your best and things still didn't turn out the way you wanted. It's okay. As long as you know you gave it your all than you should never have any shame! If you didn't give it your all, you need to look in the mirror and fix what needs fixed; never give less than 100 percent… if you do shame on you! You need to reach deep in your mind, find out what broke and you need to fix it.

Some of the greatest athletes have been on top and "BOOM" something catastrophic happens in their lives and mentally they crash. I know you think it's easy to sit here and write about how to overcome a stressful situation and keep going at the level you need to still be great at. It isn't easy by any means for anyone. It doesn't matter if you are a professional at your career or just someone regular; having something catastrophic happen is going to break you down, it's how you deal with getting back up that will define you. It's your come back that people will talk about, what do you want to define you? How you quit or how you moved forward?

I've always lived my life by the words:

"The Sun Will Come Up Tomorrow"

I'm sure there are lots of people that feel the same way; if that sun doesn't come up, then, there isn't much to worry about is there? As long as that sun comes up and is shining, even on a cloudy day, you are given another chance to better life's issues and continue on your path to your goal, keeping focused and realizing what happened is in the past and yes there may be consequences you need to deal with from your past, but regardless you need to stay focused and weather the storm! It only lasts so long. Give your mind, body and the people around you the best chance to conquer the task.

Like I said earlier, there is nothing like game day. You will experience game day jitters, they're normal. It's normal to experience those butterflies in the stomach. It's okay to throw up, it's all part of the mental preparation, it gets your adrenaline going and few ever get to experience this. Ask yourself, what will get your adrenaline going? If you are getting ready for a sporting event, maybe it's the cheerleader wearing your football jersey or preparing for the school pep rally. Maybe it's the music you are listening to while you walk into the locker room. Maybe it's that pep talk your coach is giving the team or you.

Sports, business and/or entertainment adrenaline are all similar. Closing that huge deal or stepping on Broadway for the first time, they all take preparation and how you prep is totally up to you. The feeling you get in your stomach is real, how you prep is real, you prep for you.

It's all of it! It's the love for the game.

It doesn't matter what your ambitions are, you can relate your situation to getting ready for your big game; it's symbolic of sports, whether you have participated on some level, even just by observing. Teammates, colleagues or friends: the field is your stage, your boardroom; the crowd is the people who have all eyes on you waiting for the big play; and the score is an accumulation of your effort and how you finish.

In the end, it's the work you put in all week at practice, it's the pregame preparation, it's the crowd, and it's the work in the gym. It's just as important to get your body ready for the game as is it is your mind. Your body is ready to go into battle. It doesn't matter if you are a swimmer, golfer, linebacker or an at-home mom or dad. Do you remember that engine I mentioned earlier? Your body is the engine that is about to be revved up and put through the big test. Be ready to feed your body accordingly if you want to run at full speed. Put junk in your body and your body and mind will run accordingly.

Too often, I see people not eating correctly before events, which is not what you want to be doing before practice, the big game or the board room showdown. In athletics every sport has specific eating habits prior to the big moment. You will learn what is best to feed yourself, in some cases days prior to the game, and up through pregame. A strong mind and strong body will help with conquering your goal.

You need to realize that all the work you put in at the gym over the winter or the long workouts outside in the heat of the summer were worth it. Preparing your body for the big event isn't just about eating right but it's the warm up that will not only help prevent injury but get you focused for the task at hand. Use the warm up to get your blood flowing and your heart pumping. You want to feel the goose bumps on your arms as you see fans funneling in to the stadium, the stage or the boardroom to watch you. Use the warm up to pump up your teammates or colleagues.

Your battle, as a whole, is just as important for your teammates to believe in what they can achieve as it is for you. You have to get the team to realize they are one mind and one body coming together for game day and meshing as one. This doesn't just pertain to the field, your team in the office has to get behind you and believe in you and the product. The team needs to believe in what they are doing. You each know what the others are thinking, you know their next move. It's what you have worked so hard for all year long.

10 IS IT REALLY THE END?

It all must come to an end.

The battle is over. It's time to reflect. You are bloody and sore. Your emotions are all over the place. Did you win? Did you lose? Did you do the best you could? Did your team work together as one? These questions can go on and on. Your brain is processing everything over and over right now. Your mind is running through scenario after scenario, situation after situation and play after play.

STOP!!

If you won, celebrate! Enjoy the win. Look at yourself and your team and think of the accomplishment you just achieved. It's easy to stay motivated when you have won. It's easy to reflect on a win. It's easier all the way around.

One play, one run, one misstep on stage and you could have been on the opposite side of things. You have to realize as you flaunt your win that everyone is watching, whether at a kid's soccer game or a big league ball park, people are watching how you react to your win. Some of the greatest athletes nod their heads, raise their hands and quietly walk off the field. Others are more flamboyant.

Different personalities determine how different people react. Some do it just for show and others do it for the fans. I would always suggest that keeping it classy wins above all.

If you are a winner, people are out to knock you off the top of the hill. It's harder to be knocked off the hill when you keep it classy. Don't give others a reason to hate you. Don't get me wrong, you will be hated for winning anyways, but being a sore winner only gives others a reason to want you to fail and to be knocked off that hill even more. Be humble and appreciative of your teammates and the people who have helped you get there, remember earlier I said that everyone needs help achieving their goals, you didn't do it alone.

Too often, I see athletes sit and go over all the mistakes they made (even if they won). It's okay to do that, don't get me wrong. You have to learn from your mistakes, but give yourself time to digest the win first. Reflect on your mistakes in the next day or two. Letting your mind and body decompress is so important in the learning process; it makes you better.

Everyone wants to better themselves, even after a win. You are human, everyone makes mistakes! Mentally, as you go over each play you are learning from your mistakes. Learn from them! Don't beat yourself up too badly. First of all, they are in the past so no matter how much sulking you do, nothing is going to change the outcome.

Build on those mistakes to hone your skills to become that great athlete, entertainer or entrepreneur. You are learning every day, every practice, and every game you digest a little more information and things click and are a little clearer in your mind. Sometimes as you grow as an athlete, entertainer, entrepreneur, young or old, you learn and things just seem to flow; it's like the blinders are taken off and you can see the whole world in a different way.

But, if you are on the losing end of things it's harder to remove those blinders.

Let's walk over and talk with the losers. When I talk with athletes, business men and women or anyone setting a goal, that have been on the losing end, as a motivator the first thing I teach them is to realize,

 "IT'S IN THE PAST."

No matter how much time you spend dwelling on the game or a specific play, the outcome will still be the same. Your next few moments are key to your success, it's how people deal with a loss that sets them apart. Losing a game, a potential customer, and or contract is a disappointment either way.

If you're on the losing end of an event, it will and can be mentally draining. There will be times you will question what you are doing and if you can keep going. This is where you need to bring your mind down a few notches and let things sink in.

Even athletes on the winning side of things, will sit and over-analyze every move, that's fine but give your mind a rest; you just went through a battle. Give yourself and your mind time to breathe. Give yourself time to calculate all that just happened. It's important to evaluate your actions on a clear mind. You are highly emotional and could dwell on one specific play that you may think was the one play that might have cost you the game.

It's not about that one play. Focus on the entire game. Look from the beginning to the end in what you can do to better yourself. Maybe it's staying more focused; it could be you need better endurance; it could even be working better as a team. On the losing end, it generally isn't one specific person's fault. It's always easy to find a scapegoat to blame and that is not uncommon from peewee to pros. Even in big meetings where a big deal was lost, the minds and emotions run the same as in a big game. You analyze every word that was said, every display and you wonder what happened.

As a motivator, I like to teach people that this is the perfect time to be the team leader and keep a clear head. When you feel you just don't have it in you to be the team's cheerleader, fight to keep the spirit up. It's hard, I know, but remember the event is in the past, paint over it in your mind and set the next micro goal. Make that goal part of what you will achieve in the next meeting or on the field. It's easy to point fingers after a loss but doing that only brings team spirit down. The mistakes you or your teammates have made will weigh heavy enough on the people who made them. Build off those mistakes to generate positive energy for the team and yourself. That energy, soon enough, will build some W's in the win column.

I have always said you have to be a good loser to be a good winner.

11 ONCE IT'S OVER

You get the call to come to the office, "we need to talk."

You are having trouble getting up the stairs.

You just don't move like you use to.

It's time to hang it up.

This is a life changing experience. The experience is sad but it can be exhilarating at the same time. Sad that you have to give up the thing you have grown to love and exhilarating that you are starting a new chapter in your life. Hanging up the equipment, tap shoes or briefcase is something we all face either as a professional or as a weekend athletic warrior.

As these changes come, you will face all types of emotions. It's a time to reflect on all the good times you had. This, obviously, will be a sad time in your life. It's a time of change and most people don't like change. But, you should embrace change. Take off those blinders and see the big picture.

Your family and friends are making changes also. Help each other through this important time in your life. The ups and downs everyone is facing are normal during this period of change. Look at all the positives that can come from this. Whether you're the person I described earlier working a dead end job and hating it, or the person that loves their job and can't believe they have to give it up, this change will allow you to look around and find a new you. Finding the new you will be exhilarating.

Mentally preparing for this part of your life is challenging to say the least. If you are able to see this change coming, you are one of the lucky ones. You will be able to gracefully walk away and mentally plan your departure. Being able to strategize your retirement is a key element in keeping your mental spirits high. You have the time to reflect over all the years you worked or played and you can rewind all those years in your head, sometimes playing entire games or boardroom deals or maybe specific plays over and over, until you are able to digest the need to move on.

How do you go from what seems like 100 mph to sitting at a red light?

In earlier chapters I spoke about gearing up your mind for battle. You trained your mind to withstand whatever was thrown at it during the game or meeting. You worked so hard to be prepared. Now it's time to retrain your mind for the next stage of life. Mentally slowing down is not only important for you but will be a big adjustment for the people around you. Friends and family are about to take this journey with you. Having you around more is challenging to your inner circle so they are adjusting also. Maybe your job had you on the road a lot and now your home; this is a big adjustment not only for you but your family.

For years, you kept a schedule that everyone adhered to and now that schedule includes you in it. This new journey everyone is going on can't be easily understood, unless someone has gone through something similar. Most don't understand what an athlete or an entertainer or business owner and his or her family has put themselves through over the years. When you break down the big change, think about the calm of not being on the cutting block or up for trade or changing teams to get more playing time. You and your family have the security of calling home, "home."

People mentally prepare themselves for each phase of their lives. Some phases are easier to deal with than others but regardless it's a new chapter.

In extreme cases your career may have been abruptly ended entirely too early. Maybe it's an injury or the team disbands, maybe a family crisis has you focusing on that. Whatever the case, you weren't given time to digest the end in advance. Millions of things are running through your head. You just aren't ready to give it up. You might feel you have lots of game left, but your body or people in charge feel differently. Your ability to mentally adjust to the end will be extremely important. This is a defining moment in your life, how you deal with this life changing event will be important to your future.

You will obviously need time to mentally and physically

heal; allow yourself the proper time for that healing. People often ask if there is a specific time it takes people to recover from an abrupt end to their once promising career. My response is always the same, "were you in a good place mentally prior to the end?" Everyone has their own mental demons they deal with, but were you able to control those demons in your everyday life? The point is, were you in a good place mentally? Did you enjoy your life? Do you enjoy your life? If you were happy, dealing with something so catastrophic will be easier compared to if you had parts of your life that weren't so great, if that's the case than this just adds to the misery.

The steps you take in the aftermath are vital to your future success. It's easy for people to say "move on" but moving on will be up to you. I want to say, "it's up to you when you mentally move on," but at the same time, you can't sulk. Tell yourself it happened and there isn't anything you can do about it and try to move on as fast as you can.

You need to clear your closet in your mind to allow any healing to take place. Earlier, I spoke of using "the sun will come up tomorrow," as a motto; it will help you move forward in a positive way and to allow you to realize the past is in the past and needs to stay there. Learn from it and make it a positive solution to your life changes.

Physically preparing for your new life will be difficult to say the least. As you were growing up you trained at levels that were suited for your success. You grew older and you trained to keep at the top of your game, training to score that winning touchdown, score the big contract or the next big hit on the big screen.

But now, you have been put out to pasture either by your choice or not. You must train to keep in shape and keep mentally healthy, constantly preparing to reinvent yourself.

How often have you seen athletes and professionals after retirement look out of shape? Pretty often?

Do they get back on track and get back in shape? Most do. This is all part of the preparation of "I WAS." Once it's time to move on, it's also time to get your physical well-being in check. Be part of the group that doesn't allow the couch potato bug to bite them.

Mentally you have to be in a good place to allow your physical preparation to take charge. Getting out of bed to get to the gym or to go on that walk is hard and will take a strong mind to keep going.

For years you trained for specific goals. Maybe they were sports performances or closing the deal of the century, but now it's about staying in shape and keeping healthy. It's very important to get the proper training.

Find a partner to help you conquer this part of your life. Don't try doing it yourself. Whether you ask a life coach for daily support or a friend or loved one, you need that support to help keep you on track. Your ups and downs will come and go and not allowing your physical shape to get caught up in those ups and downs is so important for both your mental and physical well-being.

You might be considering this a dark moment in your life, but, is it? Or is it just the start of something so incredible? That is up to you! Obviously, it's life changing and you will have that dark period but let's take off the blinders and see what else is out there.

So many changes are happening at once and your head is spinning. If your situation was one that you were able to plan for, or whether it was abruptly brought upon for one reason or another. Regardless, you are about to learn something new. For years you have been used to waking up to a specific routine and now it's all changed.

I'm not about to tell you getting up won't be tough at times. Some days getting out of bed will be your biggest challenge. You won't be ready for the fight some days. It will seem like the sun isn't coming up and the sky is grey.

I'm here to tell you, pull open the curtains.

The sun is shining, even through the clouds.

It will be difficult and you will need to pull from all the support you have around you and use that positive energy to get you up each morning. Use your family and friends as your crutches as you learn to walk again through life.

Whether you are male or female reading this and you were used to the weight of the world on your shoulders during your heyday, now you have to look to make a new heyday for yourself.

Building your new future and setting new goals can be invigorating and can be as exciting as your old career. Keep an open mind and an open heart.

12 KEEP IT MOTIVATED

What sticks to the wall? What do you love?

Often people going through a career change are afraid to do what they love. Maybe it's an image they feel they need to keep up with, maybe it's the unknown of what the future will bring; whatever the case may be it's important to stay motivated toward your new goal.

Hopefully you were smart with your finances growing up so that now as your life takes on this new face you can focus on this next phase. Too often in situations like this people get into a new career not because they love it, but because they need to pay the bills. If this is your scenario, than you need to make the best of it until you can find something you love and what you want to do.

Which fits you?

Paying the bills or you loving it?

No one is here to sugar coat this transition. There is no doubt that where you stand financially will determine your next move and that's okay. Learning to adjust to a specific lifestyle, no doubt could be the hardest thing to do. Wanting to do what you love may be secondary to what you have to do to keep your lifestyle at a certain level and in some cases you may need to adjust your lifestyle to accommodate the changes you are going through.

Taking this next step in the journey of life and finding out what you are going to be is a huge accomplishment. It could be like scoring the big touchdown, putting on the best performance of your life or closing that huge deal.

Let's say you love to cook and you want to be a chef but realize you don't plan on working in the kitchen. Maybe you focus on culinary classes and possibly owning your own restaurant. Learning something new is refreshing to your mind and spirit.

This is your chance to look at yourself in the mirror, clinch your fist and let the world hear you roar. I feel sorry for the people who wake up every morning, put on their clothes and pull themselves to their jobs. They look at the clock every few minutes waiting for that time to punch out. Day in and day out they do this, while day dreaming of wanting something better.

What makes you different than the average person is that you are ready to make a change or you were pushed into making a change. Either way you get that chance so many wish for. Don't throw it away. So many people wake up every morning wanting to be someone or something else. Embrace what you have been given.

ANOTHER CHANCE!

Mentally telling yourself it's okay to do what you love, will be harder, than you may think.

You already have so much on your mind, that you are feeling overwhelmed and now you have to take on one more stressor. As I stated before look at yourself in the mirror and tell yourself you are going to be great and keep doing that, until you truly feel it.

Mentally, you need to build yourself up at a time that's the toughest to go through. Life is throwing you a curveball and backing out of the batter's box isn't an option. Stand in there and take a swing. You might strike out over and over but at some point you will hit that homerun that changes everything.

That is the play you are looking for, that one thing that keeps you going. It might be career-related it might be family-related. Whatever it is, look for it and cherish it. Build off of it. Make it the new foundation to your success.

Are you prepared to not allow yourself to become that couch potato?

Don't allow yourself to fall into the rut.

Physically, you are about to enter into a new phase of your life. Your body will be going through changes. Your mind will be going through changes and everyone around you will be going through changes. Everyone is learning to adapt all at the same time. It will take some getting used to, but over time you will learn a new training method and will settle into your new you.

I Will, I Was, I Am

CONCLUSION

Life is about dreaming dreams, setting goals, modifying them and ultimately achieving success. It's about finding yourself and working hard to accomplish whatever you set out to accomplish. Sports, careers, lifetime achievements...they all come down to one thing: how high you set the bar and how hard you work for them.

Sure, along the way you'll face bumps, ups, downs and curveballs. But, what matters is how you adapt and how you persevere.

Think of your childhood dreams, turn them into goals, set a few micro-goals and make it happen. Understand that ultimately, it's you who will decide how far you go. Remember to be a realist, to surround yourself with support and to be your own biggest cheerleader.

By reading this book, you've taken the first step. Remember the lessons and steps I've outlined to heart and go for it.

You're ready for the journey. You can do it. Whatever

course adjustments you face along the way, keep pressing forward. Most of all, remember: love the NEW YOU!

Jason Jean

ABOUT THE AUTHOR

Jason is a successful athlete, entrepreneur, life coach, motivator, husband and father of two daughters, based in Central Pennsylvania. Since a young age, Jason has been about motivation and, after successfully coaching other athletes and business owners, he felt it was time to put pen to paper and show others they can set goals and achieve those goals. Be sure to pick up Jason's other motivational book, "Life's Tool Belt."